HARMONY THROUGH FOOD: AN AYURVEDIC JOURNEY

Welcome to "Harmony Through Food: An Ayurvedic Journey." This book is a gateway to the profound wisdom of Ayurveda, a 5,000-year-old holistic healing system that emphasizes the significance of balanced nutrition for overall well-being. Here, we explore the Ayurvedic diet, delve into the principles of the three doshas, and present a collection of pure Ayurvedic recipes to align your diet with your body's natural rhythms.

Ayurveda, rooted in the idea of individual constitution and the balance of mind, body, and spirit, is deeply entwined with the concept that food is medicine. This book serves as a guide to help you embrace the healing properties of food and foster equilibrium through the wisdom of Ayurvedic nutrition.

TABLE OF CONTENTS

This book aims to serve as a comprehensive guide, offering not only insights into the Ayurvedic philosophy but also practical applications through a collection of wholesome and healing recipes tailored to balance the doshas and foster well-being.

CHAPTER 1: INTRODUCTION TO AYURVEDA AND THE AYURVEDIC DIET

Welcome to the foundational chapter of our journey into the world of Ayurveda, an ancient science that illuminates the intricate balance between mind, body, and spirit. Ayurveda, the "science of life," not only offers a lens into holistic well-being but also unveils the profound connection between food and health.

In this chapter, we embark on an exploration of Ayurveda and the Ayurvedic diet, diving into the foundational principles that have guided generations toward health, harmony, and vitality. Ayurveda views each individual as a unique microcosm, influenced by the elements of nature and governed by their inherent constitution, known as doshas.

At its core, Ayurveda emphasizes the concept of balance, not just in the diet but in all aspects of life. The Ayurvedic diet is not a mere list of foods; it's a philosophy, a way of nourishing the body and soul. Understanding this ancient wisdom can empower us to make conscious, informed choices about what we consume, when we consume it, and how it affects us on a physical and energetic level.

Join us on this enlightening journey through Ayurveda, where we'll uncover the principles that underpin the Ayurvedic diet, explore the significance of food as medicine, and discover how this profound knowledge can revolutionize our approach to nutrition and overall well-being. Through the lens of Ayurveda, we'll witness the transformative power of harmonizing our diet with the natural rhythms of our bodies.

Let's delve into the essence of Ayurveda and the Ayurvedic diet to embrace a lifestyle that fosters balance, vitality, and a deeper connection to the nourishing powers of food.

Understanding The Principles Of Ayurveda:

Ayurveda, often termed the "science of life," is a holistic and ancient healing system that originates from the Indian subcontinent. Its principles stem from an intricate understanding of the human body, mind, and spirit, emphasizing the intimate connection between the individual and the surrounding environment. At the core of Ayurveda lies the belief that a balanced and harmonious state of being is crucial for overall health and well-being.

1. **The Five Elements:** Ayurveda is deeply rooted in the concept of the five elements—earth, water, fire, air, and ether—known as "Pancha Mahabhutas." These elements form the building blocks of the universe and are mirrored in the human body. Each individual possesses a unique combination and proportion of these elements, influencing their constitution or "prakriti."

2. **The Three Doshas:** Ayurveda categorizes human constitutions into three primary energy forces or

"doshas": Vata, Pitta, and Kapha. These doshas govern various physiological and psychological functions and are derived from the five elements.

- **Vata:** Comprised of air and ether, Vata governs movement, creativity, and communication.
- **Pitta:** Dominated by fire and a bit of water, Pitta controls metabolism, digestion, and cognitive abilities.
- **Kapha:** Formed by earth and water, Kapha oversees structure, stability, and emotional balance.

3. **The Importance of Balance:** According to Ayurveda, disease and discomfort arise when the doshas are imbalanced. The aim is to maintain a harmonious equilibrium among the doshas, as this equilibrium signifies good health, while imbalance leads to illness and distress.

4. **Individualized Approach:** Ayurveda recognizes that each person is unique. Understanding one's dosha constitution and imbalances is key to tailoring diet, lifestyle, and healing practices to restore balance. An individual's diet, daily routines, and activities are prescribed based on their predominant dosha.

5. **The Role of Food and Digestion:** Food is considered medicine in Ayurveda. It's not just about the nutrients but also the qualities and impact of food on the doshas. The way food is cooked, when it's consumed, and the combination of different foods significantly influences the body's balance.

6. **Healing Modalities:** Alongside diet and lifestyle adjustments, Ayurveda utilizes various healing practices such as herbal medicine, yoga, meditation, detoxification, and specific therapies to restore balance and alleviate ailments.

Understanding these principles allows individuals to comprehend their unique constitution and make informed choices that support their overall well-being. It's an approach that goes beyond the symptomatic treatment of illness, focusing on preventing imbalances and nurturing health from within.

Example in Daily Life: Consider a person with a fiery temperament, prone to overheating, and displaying strong leadership qualities. Ayurveda attributes these traits to a Pitta dominance, aligned with the fire element. Balancing this dosha involves incorporating cooling foods and practices.

The Concept Of The Ayurvedic Diet And Its Benefits:

The Ayurvedic diet embodies the belief that food is not just sustenance; it is medicine. It revolves around the idea of eating in accordance with your dosha, season, and individual constitution.

1. **Eating According to Dosha:** The Ayurvedic diet prescribes foods that balance one's dosha. For instance, a Vata-balancing diet might include warm, nourishing foods like cooked grains, root vegetables, and warming spices.

Example in Daily Life: An individual with a predominant Pitta dosha, prone to experiencing acidity or irritability, may benefit from cooling foods like sweet fruits, fresh vegetables, and grains to pacify the fiery nature of Pitta.

2. **Embracing Six Tastes:** Ayurveda recommends including six tastes—sweet, sour, salty, bitter, pungent, and astringent—in every meal for a balanced diet and to satisfy the body's nutritional needs.

Example in Daily Life: A meal might include rice (sweet), lemon (sour), a pinch of salt (salty), leafy greens (bitter), a hint of chili (pungent), and legumes (astringent).

3. **Seasonal Eating:** Ayurveda emphasizes consuming

foods in accordance with the season to maintain balance. For instance, lighter foods in summer and more grounding, warming foods in winter.

Example in Daily Life: During winter, one might include more hearty soups, root vegetables, and warming spices like ginger and cinnamon to align with the body's seasonal needs.

By aligning our diets with the principles of Ayurveda, we can experience improved digestion, enhanced energy levels, and a sense of overall well-being, fostering a deeper connection to the nourishing powers of food in our day-to-day lives.

CHAPTER 2: THE THREE DOSHAS: VATA, PITTA, KAPHA

Welcome to the profound exploration of the cornerstone of Ayurvedic understanding— the three doshas: Vata, Pitta, and Kapha. These doshas serve as the elemental energies that shape our individual constitution, govern our physical and mental characteristics, and influence our overall well-being.

1. **Understanding Vata Dosha:** Vata, composed of the elements air and ether, embodies the qualities of movement, creativity, and change. It's associated with the nervous system, governing bodily movement, communication, and imagination. When balanced, Vata individuals are creative, agile, and adaptable. However, an excess of Vata may lead to anxiety, restlessness, or irregular digestion.

2. **Exploring Pitta Dosha:** Pitta, a fusion of fire and a touch of water, symbolizes the transformative energy responsible for metabolism, digestion, and cognitive functions. Balanced Pitta individuals are sharp-minded, goal-oriented, and possess a strong digestive fire. Yet, an

aggravated Pitta may manifest as irritability, excessive heat, or digestive disturbances.

3. **Embracing Kapha Dosha:** Kapha, formed by earth and water elements, embodies stability, structure, and nurturing energy. It provides the body with strength, endurance, and emotional grounding. Balanced Kapha types are steady, compassionate, and possess strong immunity. However, an excess of Kapha might lead to lethargy, attachment, or congestion.

In this chapter, we'll dive deep into the distinctive characteristics of each dosha, understanding how they manifest in both the physical and psychological aspects of an individual's life. We'll explore the impact of imbalances within each dosha and how these imbalances can affect various aspects of health and wellness.

Moreover, we'll unravel the influence of the doshas on diet, lifestyle, and overall well-being. By understanding one's predominant dosha and recognizing its fluctuations, individuals can tailor their habits, diet, and daily routines to achieve balance and vitality.

Join us on this enlightening journey through the intricate tapestry of Vata, Pitta, and Kapha, as we unravel the wisdom of Ayurveda and its transformative potential in optimizing health, nurturing balance, and fostering a deeper connection to the self and the surrounding world.

Exploring Vata Dosha: Characteristics And Effects On Diet

Vata, characterized by the elements of air and ether, embodies the qualities of movement, change, and dynamism. Individuals dominated by Vata energy often exhibit a blend of creativity, flexibility, and quick thinking. However, an aggravated or imbalanced Vata can lead to feelings of instability, anxiety, and erratic digestion.

1. **Physical Characteristics of Vata:**
   - **Body Type:** Vata-dominant individuals often have a slender frame with prominent bones and joints. They might experience dry skin, cold extremities, and a variable appetite.
   - **Energy Levels:** Vata types can display bursts of energy followed by periods of fatigue. Their energy is like the wind—variable and changeable.

2. **Psychological Traits of Vata:**
   - **Creativity:** Vata individuals tend to be imaginative, creative, and quick thinkers. They possess a flair for artistic expression and often embrace change and novelty.
   - **Anxiety and Stress:** When imbalanced, Vata can lead to feelings of anxiety, nervousness, and restlessness. Overthinking and feeling overwhelmed are common challenges.

3. **Effects of Imbalanced Vata on Digestion:**
   - **Erratic Digestion:** An aggravated Vata can cause irregular digestion, leading to gas, bloating, and constipation. Vata types might experience hunger and fullness at irregular intervals.

4. **Dietary Recommendations for Balanced Vata:**
   - **Warm and Nourishing Foods:** Vata individuals benefit from warm, grounding foods. Cooked grains, root vegetables, soups, and stews provide comfort and stability.
   - **Moisture-Rich Foods:** Incorporating healthy fats and oils helps counter Vata's dryness. Nuts, seeds, avocados, and ghee are beneficial.

- **Herbal Teas and Spices:** Warm, soothing herbal teas and spices such as ginger, cinnamon, and cumin aid digestion and provide warmth to the body.
- **Regular Meal Times:** Establishing consistent meal times helps stabilize Vata energy and supports regular digestion.

5. **Balancing Lifestyle Practices for Vata:**
   - **Routine and Stability:** Vata types benefit from establishing a regular daily routine to bring stability and calmness.
   - **Gentle Exercise:** Practices like yoga, walking, and gentle stretching help ground the airy Vata energy without causing excessive strain.

Understanding the characteristics and needs of Vata dosha enables individuals to make informed dietary and lifestyle choices to maintain balance and harmony. By embracing foods and practices that pacify Vata's erratic nature, individuals can alleviate imbalances and foster a sense of stability and well-being.

Understanding Pitta Dosha: Diet and Imbalances

Pitta, a blend of fire and a touch of water, represents the transformative energy in the body, governing digestion, metabolism, and cognitive functions. Pitta-dominant individuals often display qualities of ambition, sharp intellect, and leadership. However, an aggravated Pitta can lead to excessive heat, irritability, and digestive disturbances.

1. **Physical Characteristics of Pitta:**
   - **Medium Build:** Pitta types often have a medium physique, with a well-defined, muscular frame.
   - **Warm Body Temperature:** They tend to have a slightly warmer body temperature, and their skin might be sensitive and prone to inflammation or rashes.

2. **Psychological Traits of Pitta:**
   - **Strong Intellect:** Pitta individuals possess a keen intellect, are goal-oriented, and have strong leadership qualities. They are precise, focused, and efficient.
   - **Tendency Towards Perfectionism:** When imbalanced, Pitta can lead to perfectionist tendencies, impatience, and a quick temper.

3. **Effects of Imbalanced Pitta on Digestion:**
   - **Hyperacidity and Digestive Issues:** Aggravated Pitta can cause excessive stomach acidity, leading to heartburn, acid reflux, and even ulcers.
   - **Increased Appetite or Aggravation When Hungry:** Pitta individuals might experience irritability or mood swings when hungry, as the fire element is closely tied to the appetite.

4. **Dietary Recommendations for Balanced Pitta:**
   - **Cooling and Hydrating Foods:** Pitta individuals benefit from foods with cooling properties. Fresh fruits, leafy greens, and juicy, water-rich vegetables help balance heat.
   - **Moderate Spices:** Mild spices like coriander, fennel, and mint are suitable, as they aid digestion without overheating the body.
   - **Healthy Fats and Oils:** Pitta types can benefit from moderate amounts of ghee, coconut oil, and olive oil to balance internal heat.
   - **Avoidance of Overly Spicy and Acidic Foods:** Steer clear of excessively spicy, fried, or acidic foods, as these can aggravate Pitta and lead to digestive distress.

5. **Balancing Lifestyle Practices for Pitta:**
   - **Mindfulness and Stress Reduction:** Pitta individuals benefit from stress-reducing activities like meditation, yoga, and relaxation

techniques to cool the fiery temperament.

- **Regular Mealtimes:** Having consistent meal timings aids in stabilizing the digestive fire and maintaining a balanced appetite.

Understanding the nature of Pitta dosha and embracing dietary and lifestyle practices that pacify its fiery nature empowers individuals to maintain balance and prevent imbalances, fostering a sense of coolness, ease, and harmony within the body and mind.

Embracing Kapha Dosha: Dietary Recommendations

Kapha, a combination of earth and water elements, embodies stability, nourishment, and endurance. Kapha-dominant individuals often exhibit qualities of calmness, strength, and a nurturing nature. However, an aggravated Kapha can lead to feelings of heaviness, attachment, and sluggish digestion.

1. **Physical Characteristics of Kapha:**
   - **Sturdy Build:** Kapha types typically have a solid, sturdy build with well-defined muscles and a tendency to gain weight easily.
   - **Moist Skin and Hair:** Their skin tends to be soft and moist, while their hair is lustrous and thick.
2. **Psychological Traits of Kapha:**
   - **Stability and Compassion:** Kapha individuals are known for their stability, grounded nature, and an inherent sense of compassion and empathy.
   - **Tendency Towards Complacency:** Imbalanced Kapha can lead to a lack of motivation,

attachment, and resistance to change.

3. **Effects of Imbalanced Kapha on Digestion:**
   - **Sluggish Metabolism:** Aggravated Kapha can cause a slow metabolism, leading to weight gain, congestion, and lethargy.
   - **Excessive Mucus Production:** Kapha imbalances can result in excess mucus in the body, leading to respiratory issues and sluggish digestion.

4. **Dietary Recommendations for Balanced Kapha:**
   - **Light and Energizing Foods:** Kapha individuals benefit from light, warm, and easily digestible foods. Incorporating more pungent, bitter, and astringent tastes helps balance the heavy Kapha nature.
   - **Stimulating Spices:** Spices like ginger, black pepper, and turmeric aid in boosting metabolism and balancing Kapha's heavy qualities.
   - **A Variety of Fruits and Vegetables:** Embrace a variety of colorful fruits and vegetables, favoring those with astringent or bitter tastes, as they counteract Kapha's heaviness.
   - **Moderate Amounts of Healthy Fats:** Using moderate amounts of healthy oils like mustard or sesame oil helps prevent excessive heaviness without causing imbalance.

5. **Balancing Lifestyle Practices for Kapha:**
   - **Regular Exercise:** Kapha individuals benefit from regular, invigorating exercise to stimulate their metabolism and energy levels.
   - **Active Daily Routine:** Establishing an active daily routine helps prevent stagnation and maintains energy levels.

Understanding the nature of Kapha dosha and adopting dietary and lifestyle practices that balance its heavy and nurturing nature assists individuals in maintaining vitality, preventing imbalances, and fostering a sense of lightness and energy within the body and mind.

CHAPTER 3: BALANCING YOUR DOSHAS THROUGH FOOD

This chapter is a guide to harnessing the transformative power of food to attain doshic balance according to the principles of Ayurveda. It explores how food—its taste, quality, and timing—plays a crucial role in harmonizing the doshas, promoting health, and preventing imbalances.

1. **Understanding Dosha Imbalances:** This section delves into the signs and symptoms of dosha imbalances. It outlines how diet-related factors can contribute to Vata, Pitta, or Kapha excesses, leading to physical, emotional, and mental disharmony.
2. **Principles of Doshic Balancing:** This part details the doshic needs and how to balance them through dietary choices. It explains the specific tastes (sweet, sour, salty, bitter, pungent, and astringent) that pacify or aggravate each dosha, offering a practical understanding for personalized diet adjustments.
3. **Benefits in Present Life Culture:**

- **Stress Reduction and Mindful Eating:** In our modern, fast-paced culture, stress and erratic eating habits are prevalent. This chapter introduces the concept of mindful eating aligned with Ayurvedic principles. It emphasizes the importance of a relaxed, mindful approach to eating, allowing individuals to connect with their food and eating habits to support doshic balance.
- **Personalized Nutrition and Health:** With the growing interest in personalized nutrition and holistic well-being, Ayurvedic principles offer an individualized approach to health. This chapter advocates tailoring diets to suit individual constitutions, promoting overall health and preventing diseases caused by dosha imbalances.
- **Preventing Lifestyle-Induced Ailments:** The incorporation of Ayurvedic dietary wisdom aids in preventing lifestyle-induced ailments like indigestion, stress-related disorders, and obesity. It encourages a shift towards a more conscious and balanced approach to eating, thus promoting wellness and longevity.
- **Dietary Adaptations for Busy Lifestyles:** Recognizing the demands of modern life, this chapter offers practical strategies for integrating Ayurvedic dietary principles into a busy lifestyle. It suggests simple yet effective changes that individuals can adopt without disrupting their daily routine.
- **Harmonizing Technology-driven Lives:** In a culture heavily driven by technology, this chapter highlights the importance of balancing the doshas to counteract the imbalances caused by excessive screen time, irregular sleep patterns, and mental stress, proposing diet as a means to restore equilibrium.

This chapter serves as a bridge between the ancient wisdom of Ayurveda and the challenges of contemporary life, illustrating the practical relevance and benefits of adopting Ayurvedic dietary practices to attain doshic balance and promote overall wellness in our present cultural context.

Customizing your diet based on your dominant dosha involves tailoring food choices to harmonize your unique constitution, promoting balance and well-being. Understanding your dominant dosha—Vata, Pitta, or Kapha—allows for personalized dietary adjustments that support your body's natural tendencies and prevent imbalances.

1. **Identifying Your Dominant Dosha:**
   - Understanding your dosha involves recognizing physical, mental, and emotional traits that align with Vata, Pitta, or Kapha characteristics. Online quizzes or consultation with an Ayurvedic practitioner can help identify your primary dosha.
2. **Vata-Pacifying Diet:**
   - **Warm and Nourishing Foods:** Vata individuals benefit from warming, grounding foods like cooked grains (oats, rice), root vegetables, and soups that provide stability and comfort.
   - **Moisture-Rich Foods:** Incorporating healthy fats (nuts, seeds, avocados) helps counter Vata's dryness, while cooked fruits and warm beverages offer nourishment.
3. **Pitta-Soothing Diet:**
   - **Cooling and Hydrating Foods:** Pitta individuals thrive on cooling foods like sweet fruits, leafy greens, and juicy, water-rich vegetables that counteract heat.
   - **Moderate Spices and Oils:** Mild spices (coriander, fennel) and moderate amounts of healthy oils (ghee, coconut) support digestion without aggravating internal heat.

4. **Kapha-Balancing Diet:**
   - **Light and Energizing Foods:** Kapha types benefit from light, warm, and easily digestible foods like pungent vegetables, bitter greens, and astringent fruits that counteract heaviness.
   - **Stimulating Spices and Exercise:** Spices (ginger, black pepper) and moderate exercise stimulate metabolism, preventing stagnation.
5. **Balanced Eating Habits for All Doshas:**
   - **Mindful Eating and Regular Meals:** Regardless of dosha, embracing mindful eating and having consistent meal times supports digestion and promotes a balanced appetite.
   - **Adapting to Seasonal Changes:** Adjusting diet according to the seasons ensures harmony with environmental changes, helping prevent imbalances.
6. **Individualized Food Choices:**
   - Ayurveda encourages adapting your diet based on the specific needs of your dosha, but it also acknowledges that everyone is unique. Some may have dual dosha dominance or varying imbalances, requiring individualized attention.

Customizing your diet based on your dominant dosha isn't a one-size-fits-all approach. It's a tailored adjustment that considers your unique constitution, promoting balance and well-being by making conscious food choices aligned with your body's natural tendencies. This personalized approach fosters a deeper connection to your body, aiding in preventing imbalances and nurturing overall health.

Using food to pacify imbalances and achieve harmony in Ayurveda involves leveraging specific dietary adjustments to address excesses or deficiencies in the doshas—Vata, Pitta, or Kapha. When a dosha becomes aggravated, it can lead to various physical, emotional, or mental disturbances. Here's how food choices can be tailored to restore balance:

1. **Understanding Imbalances:**
   - Recognizing the signs of doshic imbalances is crucial. These can manifest as physical symptoms (such as digestive issues, skin problems, or fatigue) or emotional imbalances (like irritability, stress, or anxiety).
2. **Pacifying Imbalanced Doshas:**
   - **Vata Imbalance:** When Vata is high, favoring warm, nourishing, and grounding foods is vital. Cooked grains, root vegetables, and moist foods help pacify Vata's dryness and instability.
   - **Pitta Imbalance:** For aggravated Pitta, cooling and hydrating foods like sweet fruits, leafy greens, and moderate spices assist in reducing excess heat and acidity.
   - **Kapha Imbalance:** To balance aggravated Kapha, opting for light, stimulating, and pungent foods aids in counteracting the heaviness and stagnation associated with Kapha.
3. **Tastes and Their Effects:**
   - Ayurveda uses the six tastes—sweet, sour, salty, bitter, pungent, and astringent—to balance doshic imbalances. Each taste has specific effects on the doshas and can be used to restore harmony.
4. **Creating Harmony with Opposite Qualities:**
   - Utilizing the principle of opposites, Ayurveda recommends consuming foods with opposite qualities to those of the aggravated dosha. For example, for a heated Pitta imbalance, favoring cooling foods helps restore balance.

5. **Moderation and Food Combinations:**
   - Ayurveda emphasizes moderation in food intake, as excessive consumption can further imbalance the doshas. Additionally, combining foods thoughtfully to support digestion and nutrient absorption is crucial for maintaining balance.
6. **Seasonal Adaptations:**
   - Adjusting your diet to match seasonal changes helps prevent imbalances. For instance, favoring lighter, warmer foods in colder months and cooling, hydrating foods in hotter weather supports harmony with nature.
7. **Lifestyle and Eating Habits:**
   - Alongside dietary adjustments, incorporating lifestyle habits such as mindful eating, regular meal times, and stress reduction practices complements the process of pacifying imbalances and achieving harmony.

Using food as a tool to pacify doshic imbalances and restore harmony is a fundamental aspect of Ayurveda. By making informed food choices aligned with the specific needs of your body, you can address imbalances, foster equilibrium, and promote overall well-being.

CHAPTER 4: AYURVEDIC COOKING TECHNIQUES AND INGREDIENTS

This chapter serves as a gateway to embracing Ayurvedic principles in your culinary practices by understanding specific cooking techniques, ingredients, and their impact on health and doshic balance.

1. **Cooking Techniques for Balance:**
   - **Gentle Cooking Methods:** Ayurveda recommends gentle cooking methods like steaming, boiling, and sautéing over high heat. These methods retain the natural qualities and nutrients of foods without altering their constitution.
   - **Tempering and Spices:** The technique of tempering spices in ghee or oil not only enhances flavors but also helps unlock the therapeutic properties of spices, making them more bioavailable and digestible.
2. **Balancing Ingredients:**

- **Spices and Herbs:** Incorporating specific spices and herbs based on their tastes and qualities can balance doshas. For instance, cooling spices like fennel or coriander for Pitta, or warming spices like ginger for Vata imbalances.
- **Healthy Oils and Fats:** Using nourishing oils like ghee, coconut oil, or sesame oil in moderate amounts supports digestion and balances doshas.

3. **Integrating Ayurvedic Cooking in Day-to-Day Life:**
   - **Meal Planning:** Incorporate Ayurvedic principles in meal planning. For instance, adjusting meals based on the dominant dosha or considering seasonal changes in food choices.
   - **Mindful Cooking:** Cultivate mindfulness while cooking. Enjoy the process and infuse your dishes with positive energy, known as 'prana,' which enhances their nourishing qualities.

4. **Benefits in Daily Life:**
   - **Improved Digestion:** Adapting gentle cooking techniques and using appropriate spices aids digestion, reducing the likelihood of digestive discomfort.
   - **Enhanced Nutrient Absorption:** Proper cooking methods ensure the preservation of nutrients, promoting their absorption and utilization by the body.
   - **Supporting Doshic Balance:** By selecting ingredients and using cooking techniques that balance the doshas, individuals can maintain a harmonious state of health.

5. **Practical Applications:**
   - **Cooking Rituals:** Infuse your cooking with intention and gratitude. Taking a moment to appreciate and infuse positive energy into your

meals can enhance their nourishing qualities.
- **Menu Adaptations:** Adjust your menu to accommodate the changing seasons or to address any doshic imbalances you might be experiencing.

Embracing Ayurvedic cooking techniques and ingredients in your day-to-day life offers numerous benefits by promoting digestion, supporting doshic balance, and enhancing the overall nourishing qualities of your meals. By incorporating these principles into your cooking routine, you foster a deeper connection to the healing properties of food and its impact on your well-being.

Incorporating Ayurvedic Spices, Herbs, And Ingredients

1. **Balancing Spices and Herbs:**
   - **Cumin:** Balances all three doshas, aids digestion, and reduces gas. Sprinkle it on cooked vegetables or use it in spice blends.
   - **Coriander:** Cooling for Pitta, it supports digestion and detoxification. It's versatile and can be added to various dishes.
   - **Turmeric:** Known for its anti-inflammatory properties, it balances Kapha and supports liver health. Use it in curries, soups, or golden milk.
   - **Ginger:** Pacifies Vata and Kapha, aids digestion, and warms the body. Use it in teas, stir-fries, or as a digestive aid.
   - **Cinnamon:** Helps balance Kapha, supports digestion, and balances blood sugar. Sprinkle it on oatmeal, in teas, or baked goods.
2. **Daily Incorporation:**
   - **Morning Rituals:** Start your day with warm water and a squeeze of lemon to kickstart

digestion and cleanse toxins. Add a pinch of ginger or cumin for an extra digestive boost.

- **Herbal Teas:** Brew herbal teas with spices like ginger, cinnamon, or fennel for their therapeutic benefits and enjoyable flavors.
- **Spice Blends:** Prepare homemade spice blends tailored to your dosha or current needs. Store them for convenient use in various dishes.

3. **Benefits in Daily Life:**

- **Digestive Support:** Many Ayurvedic spices aid in digestion, reducing bloating, gas, and indigestion.
- **Immune Boost:** Certain spices, like turmeric and ginger, bolster the immune system, protecting against common ailments.
- **Detoxification:** Spices like coriander and turmeric support the body's natural detox processes, cleansing and purifying.

4. **Practical Applications:**

- **Cooking and Meal Preparation:** Incorporate Ayurvedic spices into your daily cooking routine to infuse your meals with their healing benefits.
- **Health Tonics:** Prepare health tonics like turmeric milk (golden milk) or ginger tea to enjoy the therapeutic properties of these spices.

5. **Mindful Integration:**

- **Understanding Individual Needs:** Tailor your spice usage based on your dosha or any specific imbalances you might be addressing.
- **Balanced Combinations:** Combine spices thoughtfully, considering their tastes and effects on doshic balance, to optimize their benefits.

Incorporating Ayurvedic spices, herbs, and ingredients in your daily life offers a myriad of benefits, from supporting digestion and immunity to aiding detoxification. Their versatile nature allows for easy integration into various dishes, health tonics, and daily rituals, making it simple to reap their therapeutic advantages while enjoying flavorful and health-supporting meals.

Ayurvedic Cooking Methods For Optimal Health Benefits

Ayurvedic cooking methods focus on enhancing the health benefits of food while preserving its nutritional value. These methods aim to harmonize the doshas, support digestion, and optimize nutrient absorption. By adopting specific cooking techniques, individuals can alleviate or prevent various ailments linked to diet and lifestyle.

Cooking Methods for Optimal Health:
1. **Steaming:** This gentle method retains the natural qualities and nutrients of food. Steaming vegetables, grains, or fish keeps them moist and easily digestible.
2. **Sautéing:** Using ghee or healthy oils for sautéing allows for moderate heat cooking without damaging the nutrients. It also enhances the flavors of food.
3. **Boiling:** A simple and effective method to cook grains, beans, and vegetables, preserving their nutritional value while making them easily digestible.
4. **Tempering Spices:** This method involves heating spices in ghee or oil, unlocking their therapeutic properties and making them more bioavailable. It enhances both the taste and the health benefits of spices.
5. **Combining Ingredients Mindfully:** Ayurveda emphasizes combining ingredients thoughtfully to support digestion. For instance, mixing certain foods to enhance or counteract particular qualities (like

combining ginger with dairy to aid digestion).

Diseases Addressed by Ayurvedic Cooking Methods:
1. **Digestive Disorders:** The gentle cooking methods promote better digestion and absorption of nutrients, aiding in alleviating common digestive issues like indigestion, bloating, and constipation.
2. **Inflammation:** By using anti-inflammatory spices like turmeric and ginger in their cooking, individuals can reduce inflammation and potentially alleviate issues related to chronic inflammation.
3. **Metabolic Disorders:** The mindful choice of cooking methods and ingredients can aid in maintaining a healthy metabolism, potentially assisting in managing issues related to metabolic disorders.
4. **Respiratory Issues:** Certain cooking techniques can support the body in managing respiratory health, which can be beneficial for ailments such as allergies or respiratory congestion.
5. **Heart Health:** Adopting a diet prepared using Ayurvedic cooking methods, along with appropriate spices, can contribute to heart health by managing cholesterol levels and supporting overall cardiovascular well-being.

By altering the way meals are cooked and adopting Ayurvedic cooking methods, individuals can address or prevent various health issues linked to diet and lifestyle. These methods not only preserve the nutritional value of food but also support digestion, reduce inflammation, and aid in addressing a spectrum of health concerns.

CHAPTER 5: AYURVEDIC BREAKFAST RECIPES

This chapter introduces a variety of Ayurvedic breakfast recipes designed to kickstart the day with nourishing, balanced, and dosha-friendly meals. Each recipe is crafted to support digestion, align with doshic needs, and provide sustained energy for a productive morning.

1. **Vata-Balancing Breakfast Options:**
   - *Vata-Soothing Oatmeal*: A warm and grounding bowl of oatmeal cooked with almond milk, topped with cooked apples, a sprinkle of cinnamon, and a handful of nuts.
   - *Banana Almond Smoothie*: A creamy smoothie with ripe bananas, soaked almonds, a dash of cardamom, and a pinch of turmeric for its anti-inflammatory benefits.
2. **Pitta-Soothing Breakfast Choices:**
   - *Cooling Chia Seed Pudding*: Chia seeds soaked in coconut milk, flavored with a touch of rose water and garnished with sliced pears or berries for a refreshing start.

- *Pitta-Pacifying Avocado Toast*: Rye bread topped with mashed avocado, cucumber slices, a hint of cilantro, and a sprinkle of cumin to balance the digestive fire.

3. **Kapha-Harmonizing Morning Meals:**
   - *Warm Quinoa Porridge*: Quinoa cooked with warming spices like ginger, a touch of ghee, and a handful of dried fruits to invigorate and balance Kapha's tendency towards heaviness.
   - *Spiced Lentil Soup*: A light and spiced lentil soup with turmeric, cumin, and coriander to stimulate digestion and support Kapha's balance.

4. **Balanced Breakfast Staples for All Doshas:**
   - *Sattvic Breakfast Bowl*: A harmonious blend of cooked grains, steamed vegetables, and a dollop of ghee, offering a balanced meal suitable for all doshas.
   - *Fruit and Seed Parfait*: Layers of seasonal fruits, yogurt (or coconut yogurt for a dairy-free option), and a sprinkle of seeds and nuts for a refreshing and nourishing breakfast option.

Each recipe is carefully designed to cater to the unique needs of Vata, Pitta, and Kapha doshas, using ingredients and flavors that balance and support the individual constitution. The chapter aims to inspire a mindful and health-oriented approach to breakfast, fostering wellness and balanced energy to start the day.

Here are simple yet nourishing recipes tailored for each dosha:

Vata-Soothing Oatmeal:

Ingredients:
- 1 cup rolled oats
- 2 cups almond milk (or any preferred milk)

- 1-2 apples or pears, diced
- 1 teaspoon cinnamon
- Chopped nuts (almonds, walnuts) for garnish
- Honey or maple syrup (optional) for sweetness

Instructions:

1. In a saucepan, bring the almond milk to a gentle boil.
2. Add the rolled oats, reduce the heat, and let it simmer until the oats are cooked and the mixture thickens.
3. Stir in the diced apples or pears and cinnamon, allowing them to soften and infuse flavors.
4. Once done, remove from heat and let it cool slightly.
5. Serve in bowls, garnish with chopped nuts, and sweeten with honey or maple syrup if desired.

Pitta-Pacifying Avocado Toast:

Ingredients:

- Rye bread or whole-grain bread slices
- 1 ripe avocado
- Cucumber slices
- Fresh cilantro leaves
- Pinch of ground cumin
- Lemon juice
- Salt and pepper to taste

Instructions:

1. Toast the bread slices to your desired level of crispness.
2. Mash the ripe avocado and spread it generously on the toasted bread.
3. Layer cucumber slices on top of the avocado.
4. Squeeze a little lemon juice over the cucumber and avocado.
5. Sprinkle a pinch of ground cumin, add fresh cilantro leaves, and season with salt and pepper.
6. Serve as an open-faced sandwich.

Warm Quinoa Porridge:

Ingredients:
- 1 cup quinoa
- 2 cups water or vegetable broth
- 1 teaspoon grated fresh ginger
- 1 tablespoon ghee or coconut oil
- Handful of dried fruits (such as raisins or chopped apricots)
- Dash of cinnamon or cardamom for flavor
- Honey or maple syrup (optional) for sweetness

Instructions:
1. Rinse the quinoa thoroughly under cold water.
2. In a saucepan, heat the ghee or coconut oil and add the grated ginger, cooking for a minute until fragrant.
3. Add the quinoa and toast it for a few minutes, stirring occasionally.
4. Pour in the water or broth, bring it to a boil, then reduce the heat and let it simmer until the quinoa is cooked and the liquid is absorbed.
5. Stir in the dried fruits and a dash of cinnamon or cardamom for flavor.
6. Sweeten with honey or maple syrup if desired and serve warm.

These recipes cater to the specific needs of each dosha, offering nourishment and balance. Adjustments can be made according to personal tastes and dietary preferences.

CHAPTER 6: AYURVEDIC LUNCH RECIPES

This section introduces a range of lunch options crafted to balance and satisfy while aligning with the unique needs of each dosha—Vata, Pitta, and Kapha. These recipes provide balanced meals that support digestion and doshic balance.

Vata-Balancing Lunch Ideas:
1. **Root Vegetable Stew:** A hearty stew made with sweet potatoes, carrots, and beets cooked in warming spices like cumin and coriander, offering grounding nourishment for Vata.
2. **Quinoa and Vegetable Stir-Fry:** A light yet filling stir-fry with quinoa, colorful vegetables, and a dash of sesame oil, providing sustenance without overwhelming the delicate Vata digestion.

Pitta-Pacifying Lunch Options:
1. **Cucumber and Mint Salad:** A refreshing salad featuring cucumbers, fresh mint, and a light vinaigrette, cooling

for the fiery Pitta nature and aiding in digestion.

2. **Basmati Rice with Coconut Curry:** A coconut-based curry with basmati rice, incorporating cooling spices like coriander and fennel to balance the digestive fire of Pitta.

Kapha-Harmonizing Midday Meals:

1. **Warm Lentil Soup:** A spiced lentil soup with a hint of turmeric and ginger, offering warmth and stimulation to counter Kapha's tendency towards sluggishness.

2. **Sautéed Leafy Greens with Quinoa:** A light and nourishing dish combining sautéed leafy greens like kale or spinach with quinoa and a touch of ghee, invigorating and balancing for Kapha.

Universal Lunch Staples for All Doshas:

1. **Mung Bean Soup:** A nourishing and easily digestible soup made with mung beans, light spices, and a touch of ghee, suitable for all doshas.

2. **Balanced Buddha Bowl:** A bowl featuring a variety of cooked and raw vegetables, a source of protein (like tofu or chickpeas), and a mix of grains or seeds to offer a balanced and complete meal for all constitutions.

Each recipe is designed to cater to the specific doshic needs, providing balanced and satisfying meals that promote optimal digestion, nourishment, and energy. These lunch ideas aim to support doshic balance and foster overall well-being throughout the day.

Here are additional lunch recipes aligned with Ayurvedic principles, tailored for Vata, Pitta, Kapha, and universal dosha balance:

Vata-Balancing Lunch Recipes:

1. **Sweet Potato and Lentil Curry:**
   - Ingredients: Cooked lentils, cubed sweet potatoes, coconut milk, turmeric, ginger, and cumin.
   - Instructions: Simmer sweet potatoes and lentils in coconut milk with spices until tender. Serve with rice for a grounding meal.
2. **Vata-Soothing Veggie Stir-Fry:**
   - Ingredients: Colorful bell peppers, zucchini, and asparagus sautéed with sesame oil, tamari, and a touch of maple syrup.
   - Instructions: Sauté the vegetables until just tender, add tamari and maple syrup for a sweet-savory balance.

Pitta-Pacifying Lunch Ideas:

1. **Quinoa Tabouli Salad:**
   - Ingredients: Quinoa, diced cucumbers, tomatoes, fresh parsley, lemon juice, and a drizzle of olive oil.
   - Instructions: Mix cooked quinoa with diced vegetables, herbs, and dress with lemon juice and olive oil for a refreshing salad.
2. **Pitta-Cooling Chickpea Hummus Wrap:**
   - Ingredients: Homemade chickpea hummus, mixed greens, thinly sliced carrots, and cucumber wrapped in a whole-grain tortilla.
   - Instructions: Spread hummus on the tortilla, layer with vegetables, and wrap for a cooling and easy-to-digest lunch.

Kapha-Harmonizing Lunch Options:

1. **Warm Quinoa and Roasted Veggie Bowl:**
   - Ingredients: Roasted root vegetables, quinoa, a

> sprinkle of cayenne for heat, and a dash of lemon.
>   - Instructions: Combine roasted veggies and quinoa, add a hint of cayenne for warmth, and drizzle with lemon juice for zest.

2. **Spiced Lentil Salad:**
   - Ingredients: Cooked lentils, chopped bell peppers, red onions, and a tangy vinaigrette with apple cider vinegar and mustard.
   - Instructions: Mix lentils and veggies, toss with the vinaigrette for a light and satisfying salad.

Universal Lunch Staples for All Doshas:

1. **Balanced Dal and Brown Rice:**
   - Ingredients: Cooked brown rice paired with a simple lentil dal seasoned with cumin, coriander, and turmeric.
   - Instructions: Serve the dal over the rice for a complete protein and nutrient-rich meal.

2. **Mixed Vegetable Curry:**
   - Ingredients: A variety of vegetables simmered in a coconut milk-based curry with spices like cumin, turmeric, and ginger.
   - Instructions: Simmer the veggies in the curry sauce until tender and serve over quinoa or rice for a well-rounded meal.

These recipes cater to the unique needs of each dosha while offering a diverse array of flavors and textures. Adjustments can be made based on personal tastes and dietary preferences to best support individual constitutions.

CHAPTER 7: AYURVEDIC DINNER RECIPES

This chapter presents a collection of light and easily digestible dinner options that align with the principles of Ayurveda, aiming to support dosha harmony while offering satisfying yet gentle evening meals.

Vata-Balancing Dinner Ideas:

1. **Root Vegetable Stew:**
   - **Ingredients:** Sweet potatoes, carrots, beets, parsnips, cooked in vegetable broth with warming spices like cumin and ginger.
   - **Instructions:** Simmer root vegetables in broth with spices until tender. Serve as a nourishing and grounding stew.
2. **Quinoa and Veggie Stir-Fry:**
   - **Ingredients:** Quinoa stir-fried with bell peppers, peas, and zucchini in sesame oil with a hint of tamari.
   - **Instructions:** Sauté quinoa and vegetables in sesame oil until flavors meld. Add tamari for a

sweet-savory balance.

Pitta-Pacifying Dinner Options:

1. **Coconut and Lentil Curry:**
    - **Ingredients:** Red lentils cooked in a coconut milk-based curry with cooling spices like coriander and fennel.
    - **Instructions:** Simmer lentils in coconut milk and spices until they thicken. Serve with a side of basmati rice for a cooling and filling meal.
2. **Cucumber Mint Salad with Quinoa:**
    - **Ingredients:** Quinoa paired with a refreshing salad of cucumbers, fresh mint, and a light vinaigrette with lemon and olive oil.
    - **Instructions:** Toss cooked quinoa with the cucumber mint salad for a cooling and hydrating dinner.

Kapha-Harmonizing Evening Meals:

1. **Warm Lentil Soup:**
    - **Ingredients:** Red lentils simmered with warming spices like turmeric and ginger, served with a squeeze of lemon.
    - **Instructions:** Simmer lentils in water with spices until tender. Add a touch of lemon for zest and serve as a light, warming dinner.
2. **Sautéed Leafy Greens with Quinoa:**
    - **Ingredients:** Quinoa paired with sautéed leafy greens like kale or spinach in ghee, seasoned with a sprinkle of cumin.
    - **Instructions:** Sauté greens in ghee, then mix with cooked quinoa for a nourishing and Kapha-balancing dish.

Universal Dinner Staples for All Doshas:

1. **Mung Bean Soup:**
   - **Ingredients:** Mung beans simmered with mild spices and a drizzle of ghee, served as a gentle and nourishing soup for all doshas.
2. **Balanced Buddha Bowl:**
   - **Ingredients:** A variety of cooked and raw vegetables, a protein source (tofu or chickpeas), and a mix of grains or seeds for a complete and balanced meal suitable for all constitutions.

These dinner recipes aim to support doshic balance by offering easily digestible and nourishing options, fostering a sense of satisfaction without overwhelming the digestive system before bedtime.

Here are more Ayurvedic dinner recipes tailored for each dosha and universality:

Vata-Balancing Dinner Recipes:

1. **Squash and Lentil Stew:**
   - **Ingredients:** Cubed butternut squash, red lentils, vegetable broth, and warming spices like cinnamon and turmeric.
   - **Instructions:** Simmer squash and lentils in broth with spices until tender. Serve as a comforting and grounding stew.
2. **Gingered Vegetable Stir-Fry with Tofu:**
   - **Ingredients:** Tofu, bell peppers, snap peas, and broccoli stir-fried with ginger and sesame oil.
   - **Instructions:** Sauté tofu and vegetables in sesame oil and ginger. Serve over brown rice for

a filling yet gentle meal.

Pitta-Pacifying Dinner Recipes:

1. **Coconut Lime Rice with Tofu:**
   - **Ingredients:** Basmati rice cooked in coconut milk and lime juice, served with grilled tofu and a sprinkle of fresh cilantro.
   - **Instructions:** Cook rice in coconut milk and lime, grill tofu, and serve with fresh cilantro for a cooling and nourishing dish.
2. **Veggie Wraps with Cooling Yogurt Sauce:**
   - **Ingredients:** Grilled or roasted vegetables wrapped in whole-grain tortillas served with a cooling yogurt sauce flavored with mint and cumin.
   - **Instructions:** Fill tortillas with grilled veggies and drizzle with yogurt sauce for a satisfying yet calming dinner.

Kapha-Harmonizing Dinner Recipes:

1. **Spiced Chickpea Stew:**
   - **Ingredients:** Chickpeas cooked in a spiced tomato-based broth with hints of cayenne and coriander.
   - **Instructions:** Simmer chickpeas in the spiced broth until flavors meld. Serve for a light and warming meal.
2. **Quinoa and Roasted Veggies:**
   - **Ingredients:** Quinoa paired with roasted seasonal vegetables like Brussels sprouts, cauliflower, and carrots, seasoned with a squeeze of lemon.
   - **Instructions:** Roast veggies and serve with cooked quinoa, drizzle with a touch of lemon

for zest and balance.

Universal Dinner Staples for All Doshas:

1. **Nourishing Dal with Brown Rice:**
   - **Ingredients:** Yellow or red lentil dal seasoned with cumin, coriander, and turmeric, served over brown rice.
   - **Instructions:** Prepare dal and serve over brown rice for a complete protein and nutrient-rich meal.
2. **Balanced Veggie Curry Bowl:**
   - **Ingredients:** A variety of cooked vegetables simmered in a light coconut curry sauce served with quinoa or millet.
   - **Instructions:** Simmer vegetables in curry sauce and serve with grains for a well-rounded and satisfying dinner.

These additional recipes offer a diverse array of flavors and textures, crafted to support doshic balance and cater to varied taste preferences. Adjustments can be made based on individual constitutions for optimal dosha harmony.

CHAPTER 8: AYURVEDIC SNACKS AND BEVERAGE RECIPES

This chapter presents a diverse range of nutrient-rich snacks and rejuvenating beverages specifically tailored to support and balance each dosha—Vata, Pitta, Kapha—while offering universal options for overall wellness.

Vata-Balancing Snack and Beverage Ideas:

1. **Date and Nut Energy Balls:**
   - **Ingredients:** Dates, assorted nuts, and warming spices like cinnamon and cardamom.
   - **Instructions:** Blend dates and nuts with spices, roll into balls. These provide grounding energy.
2. **Spiced Herbal Tea (Caffeine-Free):**
   - **Ingredients:** Warm water, ginger, cinnamon, and a touch of honey.
   - **Instructions:** Steep ginger and cinnamon in hot water, sweeten with honey. It helps ground

and warm Vata.

Pitta-Pacifying Snack and Beverage Options:

1. **Cucumber and Hummus Cups:**
   - **Ingredients:** Sliced cucumbers filled with homemade hummus, garnished with fresh herbs.
   - **Instructions:** Create cucumber cups, fill with hummus, and garnish. It's cooling and hydrating.
2. **Coriander and Mint Infused Water:**
   - **Ingredients:** Fresh coriander and mint leaves steeped in cold water.
   - **Instructions:** Steep herbs in water for a refreshing and cooling beverage.

Kapha-Harmonizing Snacks and Beverages:

1. **Spicy Roasted Chickpeas:**
   - **Ingredients:** Roasted chickpeas seasoned with cayenne, cumin, and coriander.
   - **Instructions:** Roast chickpeas with spices for a light and stimulating snack.
2. **Ginger-Lemon Detox Water:**
   - **Ingredients:** Water infused with slices of ginger and lemon.
   - **Instructions:** Infuse water with ginger and lemon for a cleansing and invigorating beverage.

Universal Snack Staples and Beverages for All Doshas:

1. **Mixed Nuts and Seeds Trail Mix:**
   - **Ingredients:** Assorted nuts, seeds, and dried fruits seasoned with a touch of sea salt.

- **Instructions:** Mix nuts, seeds, and dried fruits for a balanced and nourishing snack.
2. **Herbal Detox Tea Blend:**
    - **Ingredients:** A blend of dandelion, fennel, and mint tea for a gentle detox.
    - **Instructions:** Brew the blend for a cleansing and supportive beverage for all doshas.

These snack and beverage recipes are thoughtfully crafted to cater to specific doshic needs while offering universal options to promote well-being and balance. Adjustments can be made based on individual constitutions and personal tastes for optimal dosha support.

Here are more Ayurvedic snack and beverage recipes, designed to cater to each dosha and provide a variety of flavors and health benefits.

Vata-Balancing Snacks and Beverages:

1. **Coconut Date Bars:**
    - **Ingredients:** Dates, shredded coconut, and a touch of ghee.
    - **Instructions:** Blend dates and coconut, form into bars. These provide nourishing and grounding energy.
2. **Chai Tea (Caffeine-Free):**
    - **Ingredients:** Warm water, ginger, cardamom, cinnamon, and a touch of honey.
    - **Instructions:** Simmer spices in water, sweeten with honey. This soothing tea aids in grounding Vata.

Pitta-Pacifying Snacks and Beverages:

1. **Watermelon and Mint Salad:**

- **Ingredients:** Cubed watermelon with fresh mint leaves, lime juice, and a sprinkle of rock salt.
- **Instructions:** Mix ingredients for a cooling and hydrating snack.

2. **Aloe Vera and Mint Cooler:**
   - **Ingredients:** Blended aloe vera gel, fresh mint, and a squeeze of lime juice in chilled water.
   - **Instructions:** Blend ingredients and serve for a soothing and refreshing drink.

Kapha-Harmonizing Snacks and Beverages:

1. **Turmeric Roasted Almonds:**
   - **Ingredients:** Almonds coated with turmeric, black pepper, and a touch of olive oil.
   - **Instructions:** Roast almonds with spices for a stimulating and light snack.
2. **Cinnamon and Ginger Infused Water:**
   - **Ingredients:** Water infused with cinnamon sticks and slices of fresh ginger.
   - **Instructions:** Let the flavors infuse for a warm and stimulating beverage.

Universal Snack Staples and Beverages for All Doshas:

1. **Seeds and Fruit Energy Bites:**
   - **Ingredients:** Mixed seeds, dried fruits, and a drizzle of honey.
   - **Instructions:** Blend ingredients, roll into bite-sized balls for a nutrient-rich snack.
2. **Tulsi and Lemon Herbal Tea:**
   - **Ingredients:** Steep holy basil (Tulsi) leaves with lemon slices in hot water.
   - **Instructions:** Let the flavors infuse for a soothing and health-promoting tea.

These additional recipes offer a broader range of flavors and health benefits, providing various options to support doshic balance and cater to different taste preferences. Adjustments can be made based on individual constitutions for optimal dosha support.

CHAPTER 9: SEASONAL EATING AND AYURVEDIC DIET

This chapter delves into the significance of aligning dietary choices with the changing seasons, a fundamental aspect of Ayurvedic principles. It explores how different foods and eating habits harmonize with nature's cycles, offering balance and wellness for each dosha throughout the year.

Understanding Seasonal Eating in Ayurveda:

1. **Concept of Ritucharya:** This section explains the concept of Ritucharya, the practice of adapting one's diet and lifestyle according to the six seasons—spring, summer, monsoon, autumn, pre-winter, and winter. It highlights the dos and don'ts specific to each season.
2. **Effects of Seasonal Changes on Doshas:** Exploring how seasonal variations can aggravate or pacify different doshas. For instance, how Kapha tends to aggravate during the spring season, Pitta during summer, and Vata during autumn and early winter.

Seasonal Foods and Recipes:

1. **Spring (Vasanta) Diet:** Discussing the significance of lighter, astringent, and detoxifying foods during this season. Providing recipes and meal ideas that aid in cleansing and balancing Kapha.
2. **Summer (Grishma) Diet:** Exploring cooling and hydrating foods for Pitta-balancing. Offering recipes for refreshing drinks, salads, and meals that help maintain a cool internal environment.
3. **Monsoon (Varsha) Diet:** Addressing the need for warmth and digestion-boosting foods during this season. Presenting recipes that balance digestion and prevent Kapha aggravation.
4. **Autumn (Sharad) Diet:** Highlighting the transition from warmer to cooler foods to prepare for the upcoming winter. Recipes focusing on grounding and nurturing Vata during this season.
5. **Pre-Winter (Hemanta) Diet:** Emphasizing nourishing, unctuous foods to build strength and immunity before the colder winter months. Providing recipes rich in healthy fats and warmth.
6. **Winter (Shishira) Diet:** Introducing hearty, warming, and nourishing meals to balance Vata during the coldest season. Recipes centered around soups, stews, and spices to maintain internal warmth.

Tips for Seasonal Eating:

1. **Adapting Meal Planning:** Providing guidance on adapting meal plans and recipes based on seasonal produce and climatic changes.
2. **Eating Mindfully:** Stressing the importance of mindful eating, understanding hunger cues, and savoring seasonal flavors for enhanced well-being.
3. **Holistic Approach:** Encouraging a holistic approach to seasonal eating, including lifestyle adjustments and exercise routines that complement dietary changes.

This chapter serves as a comprehensive guide, encouraging readers to embrace seasonal eating practices to achieve optimal health and dosha balance throughout the year. It offers practical insights, recipes, and tips to help individuals align their diets with the changing seasons in accordance with Ayurvedic principles.

Understanding the Seasonal Impact on Food Choices

Understanding the impact of seasonal changes on food choices is crucial for maintaining health and balance according to Ayurvedic principles. The seasons influence not only what's available but also how our bodies respond to different environmental energies. Here's a breakdown of the seasonal impact on food choices and how it contributes to our well-being:

Spring (Vasanta): Spring brings Kapha aggravation. The heavy, oily, and sweet foods of winter should be replaced with lighter, astringent, and bitter tastes. Bitter greens, berries, and pungent herbs help detoxify and balance Kapha.

Summer (Grishma): Pitta aggravation is common in summer. Cooling foods like cucumber, melons, and leafy greens are ideal. Emphasize hydrating foods, favoring sweet, bitter, and astringent tastes to counter the heat.

Monsoon (Varsha): This season can disturb digestion, so favor warm, light, and easily digestible foods. Dry and cooked foods are better than raw. Use warming spices to support digestion and prevent Kapha imbalance.

Autumn (Sharad): Vata starts to increase. Transition to warmer, grounding foods like root vegetables, soups, and stews. Embrace moist and oily qualities to counter the dryness of the season.

Pre-Winter (Hemanta): Focus on building strength and immunity. Foods rich in healthy fats, proteins, and warming spices are beneficial. Start incorporating heavier, more nourishing foods to prepare for winter.

Winter (Shishira): Prioritize warm, nourishing, and easily digestible meals. Root vegetables, grains, and herbal teas help keep the body warm and grounded. Embrace heavier, well-cooked dishes.

Adapting your diet to the seasons not only provides the nutrients your body needs but also helps counterbalance the potential aggravations of each dosha during specific times of the year. It allows for a dynamic relationship between your body and nature, promoting harmony, vitality, and overall well-being. Choosing seasonal, locally available, and freshly harvested foods maximizes their nutritional content, supporting a healthy and balanced lifestyle.

Seasonal Ayurvedic Eating Guidelines

Ayurvedic eating guidelines are vital for maintaining harmony within the body. Here are some strict do's and don'ts based on Ayurveda's seasonal eating principles:

Spring (Vasanta):
Do's:
- Embrace lighter, astringent, and bitter tastes.
- Opt for freshly cooked, warm, and easily digestible foods.
- Include bitter greens, berries, and warming spices like ginger and black pepper.

Don'ts:
- Avoid heavy, oily, or overly sweet foods.
- Limit cold and raw foods as they can further aggravate Kapha.

- Stay away from excessively heavy dairy or fried foods.

Summer (Grishma):
Do's:

- Focus on cooling foods such as cucumber, coconut, and watermelon.
- Include sweet, bitter, and astringent tastes in meals.
- Hydrate with fresh fruits, vegetables, and cooling herbal teas.

Don'ts:

- Avoid excessively spicy, sour, or salty foods.
- Limit heating foods like red meat, heavy cheeses, and excess salt.
- Reduce alcohol, caffeine, and hot, heavy meals.

Monsoon (Varsha):
Do's:

- Choose warm, light, and easily digestible foods.
- Opt for cooked and warm meals to support digestion.
- Include warming spices like ginger, cumin, and fenugreek.

Don'ts:

- Avoid raw and cold foods as they can disrupt digestion.
- Steer clear of heavy, fried, or excessively oily meals.
- Limit dairy as it can contribute to dampness and congestion.

Autumn (Sharad):
Do's:

- Embrace moist, grounding, and nourishing foods.
- Opt for cooked and well-spiced meals to counter Vata imbalance.
- Include root vegetables, soups, and stews to nourish the body.

Don'ts:

- Avoid dry, light, and raw foods.

- Limit overly astringent or bitter tastes.
- Steer clear of excessive intake of caffeine or stimulants.

Pre-Winter (Hemanta):
Do's:

- Prioritize foods rich in healthy fats, proteins, and warming spices.
- Include heavier, more nourishing meals.
- Opt for warm and well-cooked foods to prepare for winter.

Don'ts:

- Avoid cold or raw foods that may cause imbalance.
- Steer clear of dry or light meals that may aggravate Vata.
- Limit excessive intake of heavy, hard-to-digest foods.

Winter (Shishira):
Do's:

- Embrace warm, nourishing, and easily digestible meals.
- Opt for cooked dishes with root vegetables and grains.
- Include herbal teas, soups, and stews to maintain warmth.

Don'ts:

- Avoid cold or raw foods that may unsettle digestion.
- Limit excessively light or dry foods.
- Steer clear of heavy, difficult-to-digest meals.

Following these do's and don'ts helps maintain balance within the body and supports overall health during different seasons. Adjusting your diet in accordance with the season's natural changes can help prevent dosha imbalances and promote well-being.

CHAPTER 10: AYURVEDIC DIET FOR MODERN LIVING

This chapter serves as a bridge between traditional Ayurvedic dietary principles and their application in the context of contemporary lifestyles. It provides practical insights and adaptations to incorporate Ayurvedic dietary wisdom into our modern, fast-paced lives.

Understanding Modern Dietary Challenges:

1. **Adapting to Busy Lifestyles:** Acknowledging the constraints of modern life, where time for cooking and mindful eating is often limited.
2. **Processed Foods and Convenience:** Addressing the prevalence of processed, fast foods, and their impact on overall health.

Applying Ayurvedic Principles in a Modern Context:

1. **Mindful Eating in a Hurried World:** Discussing

techniques for eating mindfully even amidst a hectic schedule, emphasizing the importance of savoring meals and eating without distractions.
2. **Balancing Convenience with Health:** Offering guidance on making healthier convenience choices, such as prepping meals in advance, choosing healthier fast-food options, and utilizing time-saving cooking techniques.

Modern Ayurvedic Meal Planning:

1. **Balancing Doshas Amidst Daily Routines:** Providing tips on customizing daily meals to balance individual doshas without disrupting busy schedules.
2. **Incorporating Ayurvedic Principles into Daily Diets:** Offering suggestions on how to introduce Ayurvedic spices, herbs, and cooking techniques into everyday meals without extensive changes.

Strategies for Modern Ayurvedic Cooking:

1. **Quick Ayurvedic Recipes:** Presenting simple and fast Ayurvedic recipes that align with the doshas and suit modern time constraints.
2. **Meal Prep Ideas for Busy Weeks:** Providing meal prep strategies to support healthier eating habits throughout the week, catering to various doshic needs.

Adapting Ayurveda to Diverse Dietary Preferences:

1. **Ayurveda for Vegetarians, Vegans, and Omnivores:** Addressing how Ayurvedic principles can be applied regardless of dietary preferences, offering advice for a balanced diet within these frameworks.
2. **Addressing Common Dietary Ailments:** Discussing how Ayurvedic dietary practices can address modern

concerns like stress-induced eating, irregular meal times, and fast-food dependencies.

Implementing Mind-Body Balance in Daily Life:

1. **Dietary Routines and Stress Management:** Exploring how dietary changes can complement stress management techniques for a holistic approach to health.
2. **Integrating Exercise and Nutrition:** Suggesting ways to integrate Ayurvedic dietary practices with suitable exercise routines for a comprehensive well-being approach.

This chapter serves as a guide, translating ancient Ayurvedic wisdom into practical strategies for modern living. It offers insights on how to adapt and integrate Ayurvedic dietary principles into contemporary lifestyles, promoting a balanced, health-conscious approach to nutrition in the fast-paced modern world.

Incorporating Ayurvedic principles into contemporary lifestyles offers a holistic approach to health, balancing mind, body, and spirit. Here's a detailed overview of how these principles benefit and how to easily include them in daily life:
Benefits of Incorporating Ayurvedic Principles:

1. **Holistic Well-being:** Ayurveda promotes overall health by addressing not just symptoms but the root cause of ailments, aiming for balance in all aspects of life.
2. **Personalized Approach:** It recognizes individual differences, providing customized recommendations based on one's unique constitution and needs.
3. **Mind-Body Connection:** Emphasizing the connection between mental and physical health, Ayurveda promotes mental well-being alongside physical vitality.

Simple Ways to Include Ayurvedic Principles:

1. **Mindful Eating:** Take time to appreciate your meals. Chew slowly and savor each bite, minimizing distractions during meal times.
2. **Balancing the Six Tastes:** Include all six tastes (sweet, sour, salty, pungent, bitter, and astringent) in your meals to ensure a well-rounded diet.
3. **Daily Routine (Dinacharya):** Incorporate a daily routine that aligns with natural rhythms, including waking up early, meditation, oil pulling, and regular meal times.
4. **Seasonal Eating:** Adapt your diet according to the changing seasons, favoring foods that balance each season's predominant dosha.
5. **Herbal Support:** Introduce Ayurvedic herbs and spices like turmeric, ginger, and ashwagandha into your diet for their medicinal properties.
6. **Yoga and Exercise:** Practice yoga or exercise that suits your body type and supports balance.
7. **Stress Management:** Incorporate stress-relieving activities such as meditation, deep breathing exercises, and regular relaxation.
8. **Proper Sleep:** Prioritize a regular sleep schedule, aiming for sufficient rest according to individual needs.

Easily Adapting Ayurvedic Practices:

1. **Start Gradually:** Introduce one or two Ayurvedic practices at a time to avoid feeling overwhelmed.
2. **Set Realistic Goals:** Choose practices that align with your lifestyle and are manageable within your schedule.
3. **Seek Guidance:** Consider consulting an Ayurvedic practitioner to get personalized advice and guidance on your specific needs.
4. **Educate Yourself:** Read books, take online courses, or

attend workshops to deepen your understanding of Ayurvedic principles.

5. **Social Support:** Connect with communities or groups practicing Ayurveda for support and shared experiences.

Incorporating Ayurvedic principles doesn't necessarily require drastic changes. Small adjustments made consciously can gradually transform your lifestyle, promoting balance and overall well-being. By choosing practices that resonate with you and integrating them gradually, you can experience the benefits of Ayurveda in a way that suits your modern lifestyle.

Sustaining an Ayurvedic diet in a busy world requires flexibility and practical strategies. Here are some tips for integrating Ayurvedic practices into hectic schedules, whether you're a full-time parent, a working professional, or a busy student:

1. Simplify Meal Planning:

- **Batch Cooking:** Dedicate a day to prepare staples like grains, lentils, and pre-cut vegetables for the week.
- **Freezer-Friendly Meals:** Prepare large batches and freeze individual portions for busy days.
- **Crockpot or Instant Pot:** Utilize these for easy, time-saving cooking.

2. Embrace Convenience in a Healthy Way:

- **Pre-Cut Veggies and Fruits:** Opt for pre-cut or pre-washed produce to save time.
- **Healthy Snack Prep:** Prepare nutrient-rich snacks in advance, such as nuts and seeds mixes or homemade energy bars.

3. Mindful Eating Despite a Busy Schedule:

- **Eat Without Distractions:** Even during a short break, focus on your meal without multitasking.
- **Chew Slowly:** Chew each bite thoroughly to aid digestion and savor flavors.

4. Adjust Your Routine to Support Ayurveda:
- **Wake Up Earlier:** Aligning with the Ayurvedic concept of Brahmamuhurta, waking up earlier can facilitate a calmer start to the day.
- **Simple Dinacharya:** Incorporate basic practices like tongue scraping, oil pulling, and self-massage in your daily routine.

5. Adaptation for Full-Time Parents:

- **Involve the Family:** Encourage children to participate in meal prep or introduce Ayurvedic snacks.
- **Simplify Cooking:** Opt for simple yet nutritious meals that cater to the whole family's needs.

6. Ayurveda for Students:

- **Easy Snacks:** Keep simple, healthy snacks like fruit, nuts, or roasted seeds for energy during busy study schedules.
- **Routine Integration:** Incorporate small Ayurvedic practices like mindful breathing or short walks to de-stress during study breaks.

7. Integrating Ayurveda in Work Life:

- **Lunch Break Practices:** Use lunch breaks to enjoy balanced, well-prepared meals and take a short walk afterward for digestion.

- **Stress Management:** Practice deep breathing or gentle yoga stretches during breaks to manage stress.

8. Seek Community Support and Resources:

- **Online Resources:** Utilize digital platforms for meal planning ideas, recipes, and tips for balancing Ayurveda with a busy schedule.
- **Community Involvement:** Join groups or forums to exchange experiences and gain insights from others balancing Ayurveda with busy lives.

By embracing practical meal planning, adjusting daily routines, and simplifying practices, it's possible to sustain an Ayurvedic diet even in the midst of a busy schedule. Small, consistent adjustments that align with your lifestyle can significantly contribute to your overall well-being.

CHAPTER 11: AYURVEDIC CLEANSING AND DETOXIFICATION

This chapter delves into the profound Ayurvedic practices of cleansing and detoxification, essential elements to maintain balance and wellness. It focuses on ancient techniques for purifying the body, mind, and spirit to eliminate accumulated toxins and rejuvenate the system.

Understanding Ayurvedic Cleansing:

1. **Concept of Shodhana:** Exploring the concept of Shodhana, the cleansing process that aims to remove accumulated toxins (ama) from the body.
2. **Purpose of Cleansing:** Discussing the significance of cleansing to reestablish balance, enhance immunity, and revitalize the body's natural functions.

Principles and Techniques of Detoxification:

1. **Seasonal Detox:** Detailing seasonal approaches to

detoxification aligned with the changing doshic influences in different seasons.

2. **Panchakarma Therapies:** Exploring the five-fold detoxification therapies involving techniques like Vamana (emesis), Virechana (purgation), Basti (enema), Nasya (nasal treatment), and Raktamokshana (blood purification).

Gentle Cleansing Practices:

1. **Daily Detox Routines (Dinacharya):** Highlighting simple, daily practices to assist the body's natural cleansing process, such as tongue scraping, oil pulling, and dry brushing.
2. **Dietary Cleansing:** Discussing specific diets and food choices that support natural detoxification, focusing on lighter, easily digestible foods and herbal supplements.

Emotional Detoxification:

1. **Mind-Body Purification:** Addressing the importance of mental and emotional detoxification through practices like meditation, yoga, and breathwork.
2. **Stress Management:** Detailing techniques to release emotional stress and promote mental clarity for overall well-being.

Guidance for a Successful Detox:

1. **Preparation and Post-Cleanse Care:** Offering advice on how to prepare the body for a cleanse and ways to ease back into regular eating habits post-detox.
2. **Individualized Approach:** Highlighting the need for personalized detox plans based on individual constitutions and imbalances.

Incorporating Detox Practices into Modern Life:

1. **Adapting Traditional Techniques:** Providing ways to integrate ancient cleansing methods into contemporary schedules.
2. **Creating a Personalized Plan:** Encouraging readers to tailor detox practices according to their lifestyle, making it sustainable and effective.

This chapter aims to educate readers on the importance of Ayurvedic cleansing and detoxification for maintaining optimal health. It provides an understanding of various detox techniques, their applications, and the necessary steps to incorporate these practices into modern, busy lifestyles for holistic well-being.

Techniques And Recipes For Ayurvedic Cleansing

Ayurvedic cleansing involves a range of techniques and recipes that aid in the elimination of toxins and rejuvenation of the body. Here are details on specific techniques and recipes used in Ayurvedic cleansing:

1. Abhyanga (Self-Massage):

- **Technique:** Using warm, dosha-specific oils for self-massage, particularly sesame oil for Vata, coconut oil for Pitta, and mustard oil for Kapha. This gentle massage promotes lymphatic drainage and aids in toxin removal.

2. Svedana (Herbal Steam Therapy):

- **Technique:** Engaging in herbal steam therapy using Ayurvedic herbs like ginger, eucalyptus, or neem. This technique helps in opening the pores and releasing toxins through sweating.

3. Triphala Tea for Detoxification:

- **Recipe:** Boil water and steep Triphala powder for 10-15 minutes. Strain and drink this herbal tea daily to aid digestion and elimination.

4. Detoxifying Kitchari Cleanse:

- **Recipe:** Prepare a cleansing Kitchari using mung beans, basmati rice, ghee, and digestive spices like cumin, coriander, and turmeric. This easy-to-digest meal supports the digestive system during detoxification.

5. Detoxifying Herbal Teas:

- **Recipes:**
  - Boil water with fresh ginger, turmeric, and a dash of black pepper for an anti-inflammatory and detoxifying tea.
  - Boil water with coriander, cumin, and fennel seeds to aid digestion and reduce toxins.

6. Tongue Scraping and Oil Pulling:

- **Techniques:** Practicing daily tongue scraping to remove toxins accumulated overnight on the tongue. Oil pulling with coconut or sesame oil for a few minutes helps draw out toxins from the body.

7. Detoxifying Herbal Supplements:

- **Triphala:** A popular herbal supplement aiding in digestion and gentle cleansing.
- **Guduchi:** Known for its detoxification properties, supporting the immune system and liver health.

8. Fasting Practices:

- **Technique:** Short-term fasting or periodic fasting can aid in the body's natural detoxification process. This might include a day of consuming only warm liquids or consuming lighter meals for a specific period.

These techniques and recipes aim to aid the body's natural detoxification process, remove accumulated toxins, and rejuvenate the system. They are often employed as part of short-term cleansing practices, especially during seasonal changes, to support the body's inherent healing mechanisms and promote balance and well-being.

Nourishing Detox Plans Based On Doshas

Nourishing detox plans aligned with individual doshas involves tailoring cleansing techniques and diets according to one's predominant doshic constitution. Here's a breakdown based on the three doshas:

1. Vata Dosha:

Detox Focus: Aim for grounding and warming techniques to balance Vata's airy and light qualities.

- **Techniques:** Emphasize warm oil massages (Abhyanga) using sesame oil, gentle yoga, and warm herbal steam therapies to ground Vata.
- **Dietary Emphasis:** Opt for nourishing, easily digestible foods like cooked grains, root vegetables, herbal teas, and warming spices (ginger, cinnamon, and cumin) to pacify Vata's erratic nature.

2. Pitta Dosha:

Detox Focus: Cooling and calming techniques to soothe Pitta's fiery nature.

- **Techniques:** Incorporate gentle yoga, meditation, and cooling herbal steam therapies using herbs like sandalwood or rose petals to pacify Pitta.
- **Dietary Emphasis:** Include cooling, hydrating foods like cucumbers, leafy greens, sweet fruits, and aloe vera juice. Favor sweet, bitter, and astringent tastes to balance Pitta's intensity.

3. Kapha Dosha:

Detox Focus: Revitalizing and stimulating techniques to counter Kapha's heavy and sluggish characteristics.

- **Techniques:** Opt for invigorating exercises, like vigorous yoga, brisk walks, and herbal steam therapies with stimulating herbs like ginger or eucalyptus to counter Kapha's stagnation.
- **Dietary Emphasis:** Include light, spicy foods, incorporating bitter, pungent, and astringent tastes. Focus on legumes, light grains, and warming spices (turmeric, black pepper) to balance Kapha's heaviness.

Creating a nourishing detox plan involves applying cleansing techniques and dietary adjustments that specifically target the imbalances associated with each dosha. By using a combination of appropriate therapies and diets, individuals can support their body's natural detoxification process while addressing their unique doshic needs.

CHAPTER 12: MINDFUL EATING AND AYURVEDA

This chapter emphasizes the profound connection between conscious eating and Ayurvedic principles, highlighting the impact of mindful eating habits on overall health and well-being. It delves into the importance of not just what we eat, but how we eat, aligning with Ayurvedic teachings.

Understanding Mindful Eating:

1. **The Mind-Body Connection:** Exploring how mindful eating establishes a connection between the mind, body, and food, promoting holistic health.
2. **Sensory Experience:** Delving into the importance of savoring flavors, textures, and aromas to enhance the overall eating experience.

Principles of Mindful Eating in Ayurveda:
1. **Eating According to Doshas:** Discussing the impact of eating habits on doshic balance and providing guidelines for Vata, Pitta, and Kapha constitutions.
2. **Synchronization with Nature:** Emphasizing the

significance of eating in accordance with the natural rhythms and cycles.

Mindful Eating Practices:

1. **Slowing Down and Savoring:** Encouraging readers to eat slowly, chew thoroughly, and appreciate each bite, fostering better digestion and assimilation.
2. **Eating with Awareness:** Advising on being present during meals, avoiding distractions, and focusing on the act of eating itself.

Customized Approaches for Different Doshas:

1. **Vata Dosha:** Recommendations for grounding foods and routines to stabilize Vata's airy and erratic nature during meals.
2. **Pitta Dosha:** Guidelines for cooling and calming meals to manage Pitta's intense and fiery qualities.
3. **Kapha Dosha:** Suggestions for light, stimulating foods and practices to counter Kapha's heavy and sluggish tendencies during eating.

Mindful Eating Rituals:

1. **Gratitude and Intention Setting:** Encouraging practices such as expressing gratitude before meals and setting intentions for mindful and nourishing eating.
2. **Cleansing Practices:** Incorporating gentle cleansing practices before and after meals to support the body's natural processes.

Mind-Body Impact:

1. **Digestive Health and Emotional Well-being:** Exploring the correlation between mindful eating and improved

digestion, as well as emotional balance.

2. **Satiety and Portion Control:** Understanding how eating mindfully aids in recognizing true hunger and fullness cues, promoting appropriate portion sizes.

This chapter serves as a guide to cultivate a mindful approach to eating, aligning with Ayurvedic wisdom. It emphasizes the significance of not just the food choices but also the manner in which one consumes meals, fostering a deeper connection between food, body, and overall well-being.

Importance Of Mindfulness In Ayurvedic Nutrition:

Mindfulness in Ayurvedic nutrition plays a crucial role in fostering a deeper connection with food, promoting better digestion, and maintaining overall well-being. Here are the key points on its importance and some simple mindful practices:

1. **Enhanced Digestion:** Eating mindfully supports optimal digestion, allowing the body to properly break down and absorb nutrients from food.
2. **Connection to Food:** Mindfulness creates a deeper relationship with food, fostering appreciation for its quality, taste, and its impact on the body.
3. **Balanced Doshas:** Mindful eating helps in balancing doshas by choosing foods and practices that align with individual constitutions, preventing imbalances.
4. **Emotional Well-being:** By being present during meals, one can promote emotional balance, as eating mindfully reduces stress and promotes relaxation.

Easy Mindful Practices for Health:

1. **Mindful Breathing:** Take a few deep breaths before

eating to calm the mind and prepare the body for digestion.

2. **Gratitude Ritual:** Express gratitude for the meal, acknowledging the effort and energy put into its preparation.

3. **Engage the Senses:** Observe the colors, textures, and aromas of your meal before taking the first bite to engage the senses fully.

4. **Chew Thoroughly:** Slow down and chew each bite thoroughly, savoring the taste and texture of the food.

5. **Portion Awareness:** Be aware of portion sizes, eating until feeling satisfied, not excessively full.

6. **Mindful Cooking:** When preparing meals, focus on the process, infusing love and positive energy into the food.

7. **Mindful Snacking:** Consciously choose snacks, focusing on nutrient-rich options like fruits, nuts, or seeds, avoiding mindless eating.

8. **Appreciation and Reflection:** Take a moment after the meal to appreciate the nourishment received and reflect on how the food made you feel.

By integrating these mindful practices into daily life, individuals can foster a deeper connection with food, promote better digestion, and support their overall health and well-being according to Ayurvedic principles.

Rituals And Practices For Mindful Eating With Timings:

1. **Pre-Meal Preparation (5-10 minutes):**
   - **Mindful Set-Up:** Set an environment conducive to mindful eating, free from distractions like phones or screens.
   - **Breathing Exercise:** Engage in a short breathing exercise to relax the mind and

prepare the body for digestion.

2. **Gratitude and Intention Setting (1-2 minutes):**
   - **Express Gratitude:** Take a moment to appreciate the food and the effort behind its preparation.
   - **Set Intention:** Set an intention to eat mindfully, focusing on nourishing the body and fostering a deeper connection with food.

3. **Observing and Engaging with the Meal (5-10 minutes):**
   - **Engage the Senses:** Observe the colors, textures, and aromas of the meal, engaging the senses fully.
   - **Mindful Portioning:** Serve appropriate portions, avoiding overeating.

4. **Chewing and Savoring (15-20 minutes):**
   - **Chew Thoroughly:** Chew each bite slowly and thoroughly, savoring the taste and texture of the food.
   - **Mindful Sips:** If drinking with the meal, take small, mindful sips to aid digestion.

5. **Reflection and Gratitude (1-2 minutes):**
   - **Appreciation:** After finishing the meal, take a moment to appreciate the nourishment received and the experience of eating mindfully.
   - **Reflect:** Reflect on how the food made you feel physically and emotionally.

Importance of Mindful Eating and Consequences of Not Practicing It:

When Done Right:

- **Enhanced Digestion:** Mindful eating promotes better digestion, aiding the body in breaking down food efficiently.

- **Balanced Doshas:** Helps in balancing doshas by choosing foods that align with individual constitutions, preventing imbalances.
- **Emotional Well-being:** Reduces stress and promotes relaxation, fostering emotional balance.

When Not Practiced:

- **Poor Digestion:** Eating in a hurry or without attention can lead to poor digestion, causing discomfort like bloating or indigestion.
- **Imbalance in Doshas:** Mindless eating without considering one's constitution can potentially lead to doshic imbalances.
- **Emotional Impact:** Rushed eating might lead to heightened stress and reduced enjoyment of meals, impacting emotional well-being.

Engaging in mindful eating rituals supports optimal digestion, emotional balance, and overall health. Not practicing mindfulness during meals might lead to imbalances and discomfort, impacting both physical and emotional well-being.

CHAPTER 13: CREATING AN AYURVEDIC KITCHEN

This chapter focuses on transforming your kitchen into an environment that supports Ayurvedic principles, fostering the preparation of healthful, balanced meals aligned with individual constitutions.

Understanding the Ayurvedic Kitchen:

1. **Importance of Kitchen Setup:** Exploring the significance of a well-organized and harmonious kitchen space in promoting healthy eating habits.
2. **Aligning with Ayurvedic Principles:** Discussing how the kitchen setup can support doshic balance and overall well-being.

Creating an Ayurvedic Kitchen:

1. **Optimal Kitchen Design:** Suggestions for an organized kitchen layout, emphasizing ease of movement, efficient storage, and access to essential tools and ingredients.
2. **Selecting Cookware and Utensils:** Guidance on

choosing suitable materials for cookware and utensils in line with Ayurvedic practices, such as copper, stainless steel, or cast iron.

Kitchen Elements According to Doshas:

1. **Vata-Pacifying Kitchen:** Recommendations for warm and grounding elements, like earthy tones, to balance Vata's airy nature.
2. **Pitta-Soothing Kitchen:** Tips for creating a cooler, calming environment with lighter colors and calming elements to pacify Pitta's fiery disposition.
3. **Kapha-Revitalizing Kitchen:** Suggestions for a vibrant, stimulating kitchen with bright colors and natural light to counter Kapha's heaviness.

Stocking an Ayurvedic Kitchen:

1. **Essential Ingredients:** Detailing essential spices, herbs, grains, and legumes commonly used in Ayurvedic cooking.
2. **Fresh Produce:** Encouragement to include a variety of fresh, seasonal produce to support balanced nutrition.

Incorporating Mindfulness:

1. **Mindful Cooking Practices:** Emphasizing the importance of infusing cooking with positive energy, intention, and mindfulness.
2. **Food Storage and Handling:** Suggestions for mindful food storage practices to maintain freshness and nutrition.

Promoting Hygiene and Balance:

1. **Cleanliness and Organization:** Stressing the

significance of a clean and organized kitchen to promote overall health.

2. **Energetic Balance:** Tips on how to maintain an energetically balanced kitchen space to foster positive cooking experiences.

The chapter serves as a guide for creating a kitchen environment aligned with Ayurvedic principles, encouraging a mindful and balanced approach to food preparation and cooking. It focuses on supporting not only physical health but also the overall well-being of individuals following an Ayurvedic lifestyle.

How To Set Up Your Kitchen In Alignment With Ayurveda:

Setting up your kitchen in alignment with Ayurvedic principles involves creating an environment that supports a healthy, balanced, and mindful approach to food preparation and consumption. Here's a detailed guide on how to do it, why it's important, and the benefits it brings to both individuals and the household:

1. **Optimal Kitchen Design:**
   - **Efficient Layout:** Arrange the kitchen for easy movement, accessibility, and efficient storage of essential cooking tools and ingredients.
   - **Organized Zones:** Create distinct zones for food preparation, cooking, and storing utensils and ingredients.
2. **Selecting Cookware and Utensils:**
   - **Material Choice:** Choose cookware made of materials such as stainless steel, copper, or cast iron, which align with Ayurvedic practices and cooking methods.
3. **Balanced Colors and Elements:**

- **Vata-Balancing:** Warm, earthy tones to ground Vata's airy nature.
- **Pitta-Soothing:** Lighter, calming colors to pacify Pitta's intensity.
- **Kapha-Revitalizing:** Bright, stimulating colors and natural light to counter Kapha's heaviness.

4. **Essential Ingredients and Fresh Produce:**
   - **Stocking Ayurvedic Essentials:** Include a variety of spices, herbs, grains, and legumes essential for Ayurvedic cooking.
   - **Seasonal and Fresh Produce:** Incorporate a diverse range of fresh, seasonal produce to support balanced nutrition.

5. **Mindful Cooking Practices:**
   - **Intentions and Energy:** Infuse cooking with positive intentions and mindfulness, creating a space of nourishment and positivity.

6. **Hygiene and Energetic Balance:**
   - **Cleanliness:** Maintain a clean, organized, and clutter-free kitchen to promote overall hygiene.
   - **Energetic Balance:** Foster a positive cooking environment by maintaining an energetically balanced space.

Why Set Up an Ayurvedic Kitchen:

- **Health and Well-being:** Supporting a healthy cooking environment promotes overall health and well-being.
- **Nutritional Balance:** It encourages balanced, nutritious meals aligned with individual constitutions.
- **Mindful Eating:** A well-organized kitchen space fosters a mindful approach to cooking and eating, aiding digestion and emotional well-being.

Benefits to Individuals and the Household:

1. **Individual Health:** Supports an individual's well-being by providing balanced and nutritious meals.
2. **Family Harmony:** Encourages mindful eating practices, fostering a positive environment for the entire household.
3. **Hygiene and Efficiency:** Maintaining a clean and organized kitchen promotes efficiency in meal preparation and prevents food-related health issues.

Creating an Ayurvedic kitchen promotes a holistic and balanced approach to cooking and eating. It benefits both individuals and the household by fostering health, harmony, and a mindful connection with food.

Tools, Storage, And Organization Tips For An Ayurvedic Kitchen:

Essential Tools:

1. **Quality Cookware:** Opt for stainless steel, copper, or cast iron pots and pans, as they align with Ayurvedic principles.
2. **Spice Grinder and Mortar & Pestle:** Grind fresh spices and herbs to preserve their potency and flavor.
3. **Chopping Boards and Quality Knives:** Ensure efficient and safe food preparation with proper cutting tools.

Storage and Organization:

1. **Adequate Pantry Space:** Store dry goods like grains, legumes, and spices in a cool, dry, and organized pantry area.
2. **Refrigeration Management:** Keep fresh produce in a designated section in the refrigerator to maintain freshness.

3. **Labeling and Organization:** Label jars and containers to easily identify and access various spices, grains, and herbs.

Benefits in Life and Mood Changes:

1. **Efficiency in Cooking:** Having the right tools and an organized kitchen makes meal preparation more efficient, reducing stress and saving time.
2. **Enhanced Flavor Profiles:** Freshly ground spices and properly stored ingredients enhance the flavor and nutritional value of dishes, promoting a more enjoyable dining experience.
3. **Emotional Well-being:** A clean, organized kitchen can positively impact mood and reduce stress associated with meal preparation, fostering a more relaxed and pleasant cooking environment.

A well-equipped, organized Ayurvedic kitchen not only promotes efficient and mindful cooking but also positively influences mood and emotional well-being, fostering a more enjoyable and relaxed environment for meal preparation.

BALANCED LIVING: NOURISHING HARMONY THROUGH AYURVEDIC CUISINE

"Harmony Through Food: An Ayurvedic Journey" concludes with a celebration of the profound connection between food, well-being, and harmony. Through this exploration, we've discovered that the kitchen isn't merely a place for cooking but a sacred space where nutrition, mindfulness, and balance converge.

Key Learnings:

1. **Mindful Connection:** We've learned to establish a deeper connection with food, practicing mindful eating and mindful cooking to nurture the body, mind, and soul.
2. **Individualized Nutrition:** Understanding our unique constitutions (Vata, Pitta, Kapha) allows us to tailor diets that support our specific needs, promoting balance and well-being.
3. **Rituals and Practices:** Incorporating Ayurvedic rituals and practices—such as mindful cooking, kitchen organization, and the use of healing spices—enhances our culinary experience and well-being.

4. **Holistic Living:** The kitchen, when aligned with Ayurvedic principles, becomes a sanctuary fostering not just health but emotional balance and a harmonious atmosphere.

The Path to Harmony:

This journey has empowered us to embrace food not just as sustenance but as a pathway to harmony. By creating an Ayurvedic kitchen, infusing mindfulness into cooking and eating, and embracing individualized nutrition, we foster not just a healthier lifestyle but a more connected and contented way of living.

In essence, "Harmony Through Food: An Ayurvedic Journey" is a celebration of the profound wisdom that our kitchens hold, guiding us towards holistic well-being and a deeper understanding of the intricate relationship between what we eat and how it shapes our lives. It's an invitation to savor not just the flavors of our meals but the harmony and balance they bring to our existence.